COPYRIGHT

The Covid Mood
For Inquiries, call 410-903-1469
www.thecovidmood.com

Printed in USA
ISBN: 978-1-7948-2875-9
Published by Lulu Publishing

The information in this book has been carefully researched, and every reasonable effort has been made to ensure it's accuracy. The book's publisher nor creators assume any liability for any accidents, injuries, losses or other damages that might occur from it's use. You are solely responsible for taking any and all reasonable precautions when performing the activities from this workbook.

All rights reserved. No part of this book may be reproduced in any form or by any electronic means, including information storage and retrieval systems, without permission from it's author and associated publisher.

Certain graphics used in this publication are used by license or permission from the owner thereof, or are publicly available. This publication is not endorsed by any person or entity herein.

Author: Latoya Hounshell

All Images Canva

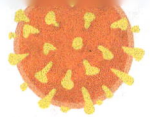

COVIDCARE

HOME SURVIVAL KIT

SAFE CARE FROM HOME DURING QUARANTINE.

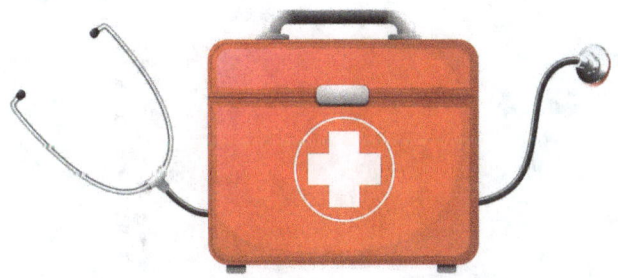

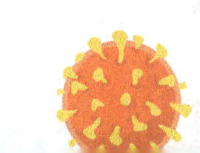

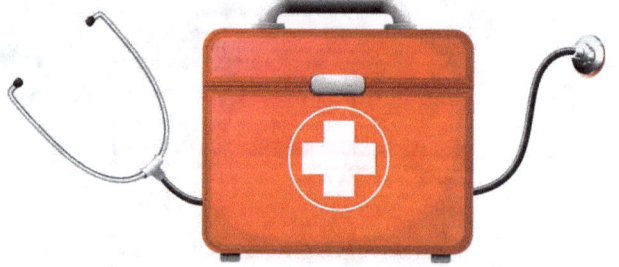

COVIDCARE

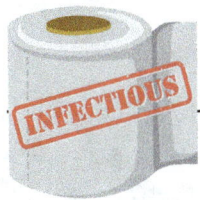

INTRODUCTION

To date of this publication, 5 million people around the world have died after being infected with the Coronavirus disease (Covid-19). Around a third of those deaths have occurred within the homes of sick individuals.

The Coronavirus Home Survival Workbook was designed to educate as many households as possible in the awareness of self-care and careful monitoring during the stages of viral infection.

This publication is also dedicated to All FRONTLINE MEDICAL WORKERS around the world, who's strength and mental agility stood the test of time against unsurmountable working conditions, while keeping in mind the greater good of the mission.

" We Are Brave.
We Have Heart..
We Are The Mission..." L.H.

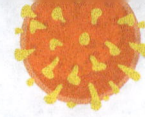

HOME SURVIVAL TIP SHEETS AND TASK GUIDE

SAFE CARE FROM HOME DURING QUARANTINE.

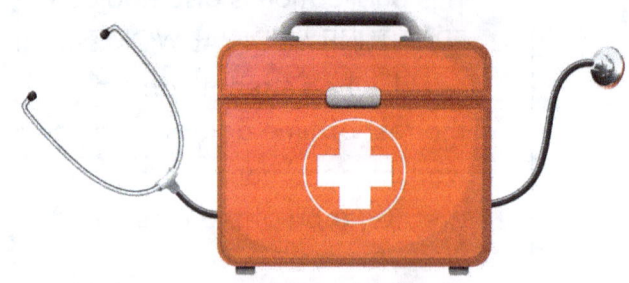

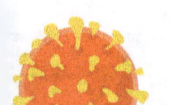
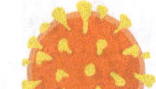
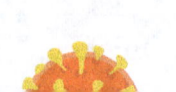

COVIDCARE

Gathering Necessary Supplies

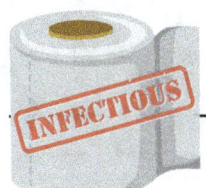

HOME SURVIVAL TIP SHEET

- [ ] You will need an automatic blood pressure cuff, thermometer & finger pulse oxygen monitor. (Can be found at local drug store, Amazon or provided by healthcare team).

- [ ] Designate one person to care for you and the other members of the household. Ensure that every person in the home wears a mask. (N95, Level 3 Mask or Double Mask)

- [ ] Use paper plates, cups and eating utensils. Dispose in a designated trash bag after every use!

- [ ] Purchase disinfectant wipes & spray, paper towels, trash bags & plastic gloves. Place items in every room where you or loved one is anticipated to touch or stay.

- [ ] Disinfect all highly touched surfaces and spray contaminated areas every 2-3 hours throughout the day to reduce the chance of viral transmission.

- [ ] **Seek Medical Attention Immediately** if your condition worsens or if your finger pulse oxygen *level reaches below 91%.*

COVIDCARE

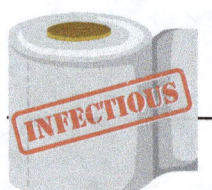

Symptom And Viral Stage Monitoring

HOME SURVIVAL TASK GUIDE

- ☐ Gather all necessary care supplies and affix corresponding door alert to your place of quarantine. Door Alert Enclosed.

- ☐ Monitor your vitals and symptoms every 2 hours days 1-4 after a confirmed positive Covid-19 Result.

- ☐ Monitor your vitals and symptoms every 4 hours days 5-7.

- ☐ Keep Calm! Hopefully you are starting to feel better. Monitor your symptoms and vitals every 8 hours days 8-10.

- ☐ Follow the warning icons located at the top left corner of your daily guide.

- ☐ Seek Medical Attention Immediately if your condition worsens. Take this guide with you to help your healthcare team.

COVIDCARE

Natural Care Remedies

HOME CARE NATURAL REMEDIES TIP SHEET

- Crack room window slightly and utilize an air vaporizer. Place vapor pads into designated spots of the vaporizer. Lavender Calming Vapor Pack Preferred.

- Teas are soothing and aid in the healing process. Boil 1 cup of water with a lemon and ginger tea bag. Add 2 drops of honey, tablespoon of turmeric powder and 1 ginger cube.

- Acetaminophen & Ibuprofen reduce muscle aches and reduce fevers. Follow the manufactures product information for correct dosage and usage.

- I recommend Zero Sugar vitamin water and Zero Sugar Body Armour which is packed with essential vitamins for an energy boost.

- Hug a pillow and practice deep slow and short breaths up to 10 times an hour as tolerated to exercise lung muscles.

- Obtain a product containing Black Elderberry Rich in Zinc, Vitamin C, Echinacea & Astragalus, which is great for immune support. Follow Product Information Usage.

These statments are not intended to diagnose, treat, cure, or prevent any disease.

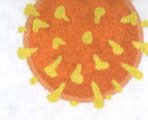

HOME SURVIVAL INFECTION REDUCTION

SAFE CARE FROM HOME DURING QUARANTINE.

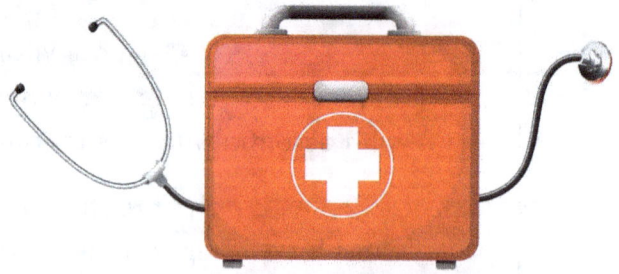

How to Wear Masks

Protect yourself and others by observing proper mask handling.

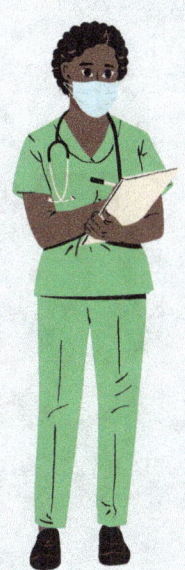

Inspect

Before putting on your mask, make sure they're clean and without damage.

Secure

Make sure your mask covers your nose, mouth, and chin.

Avoid

While wearing your mask, avoid touching it. In case you do, wash your hands immediately.

Remove

Use the ear loops when removing your mask. Don't touch the front fabric to avoid transferring viruses or germs to your hands.

How to Wash Hands

Reduce the risk of viral transmission by properly washing hands consistently through out the day and when touching high contact surfaces.

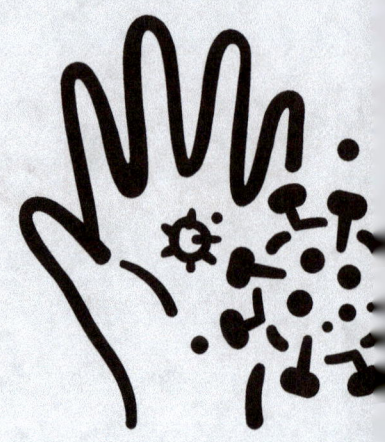

Rinse with Water

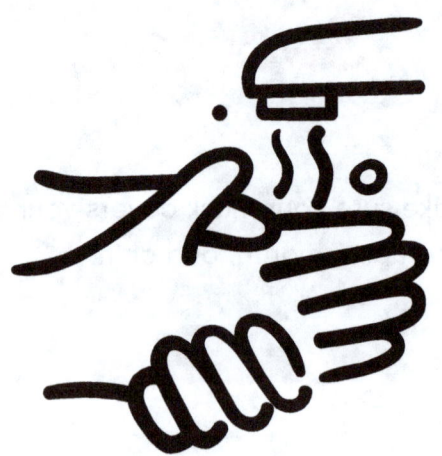

Lather with Soap

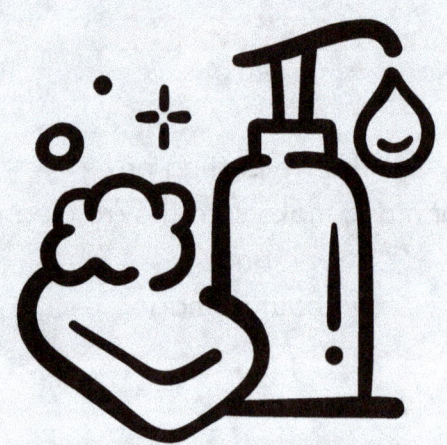

Scrub for 20 Secs

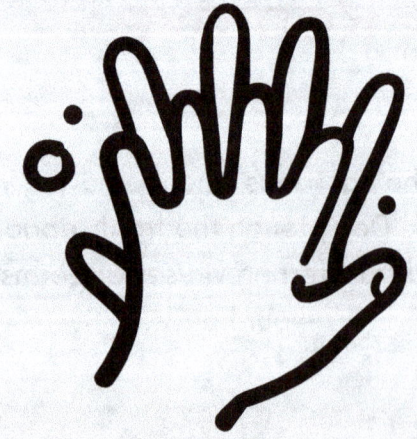

Dry Hands

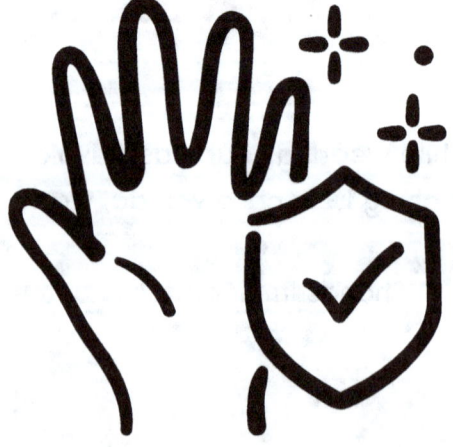

What Are The Coronavirus Disease Symptoms

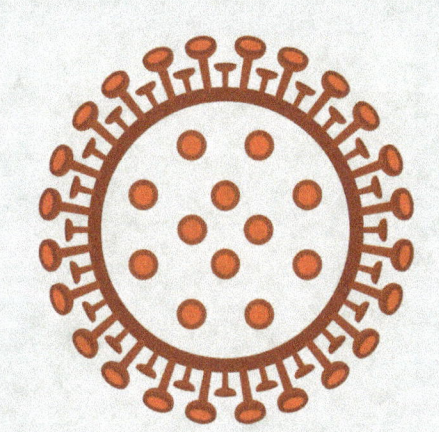

The Coronavirus (Covid-19) Displays A Variety of Symptoms that Masks Itself Like a Common Cold & The Flu.

FEVER

COUGH

FATIGUE

LOSS OF TASTE

OR

LOSS OF SMELL

Severe Headache

Body Aches & Pains

Red Glassy Eyes

Difficulty Breathing

AND OR

Shortness of Breath

HIGHLY INFECTIOUS

USE EXTREME CAUTION

QUARANTINE

DAYS 1-4

PLACE ON DOOR

HIGHLY INFECTIOUS

USE EXTREME CAUTION

DAYS 1-4

HIGHLY INFECTIOUS

SYMPTOMS & VITAL SIGNS WORKSHEETS

QUARANTINE

DAYS 1-4

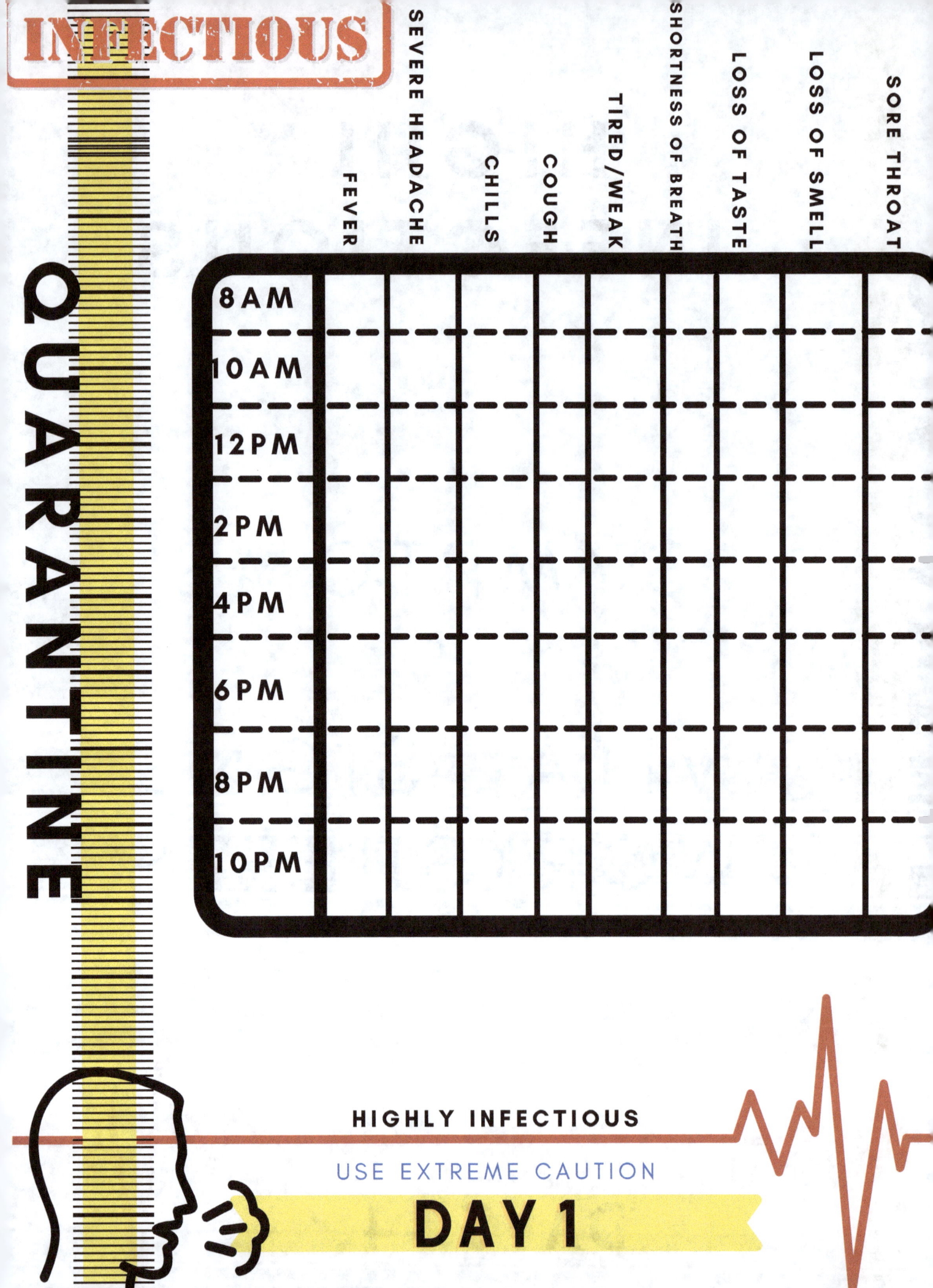

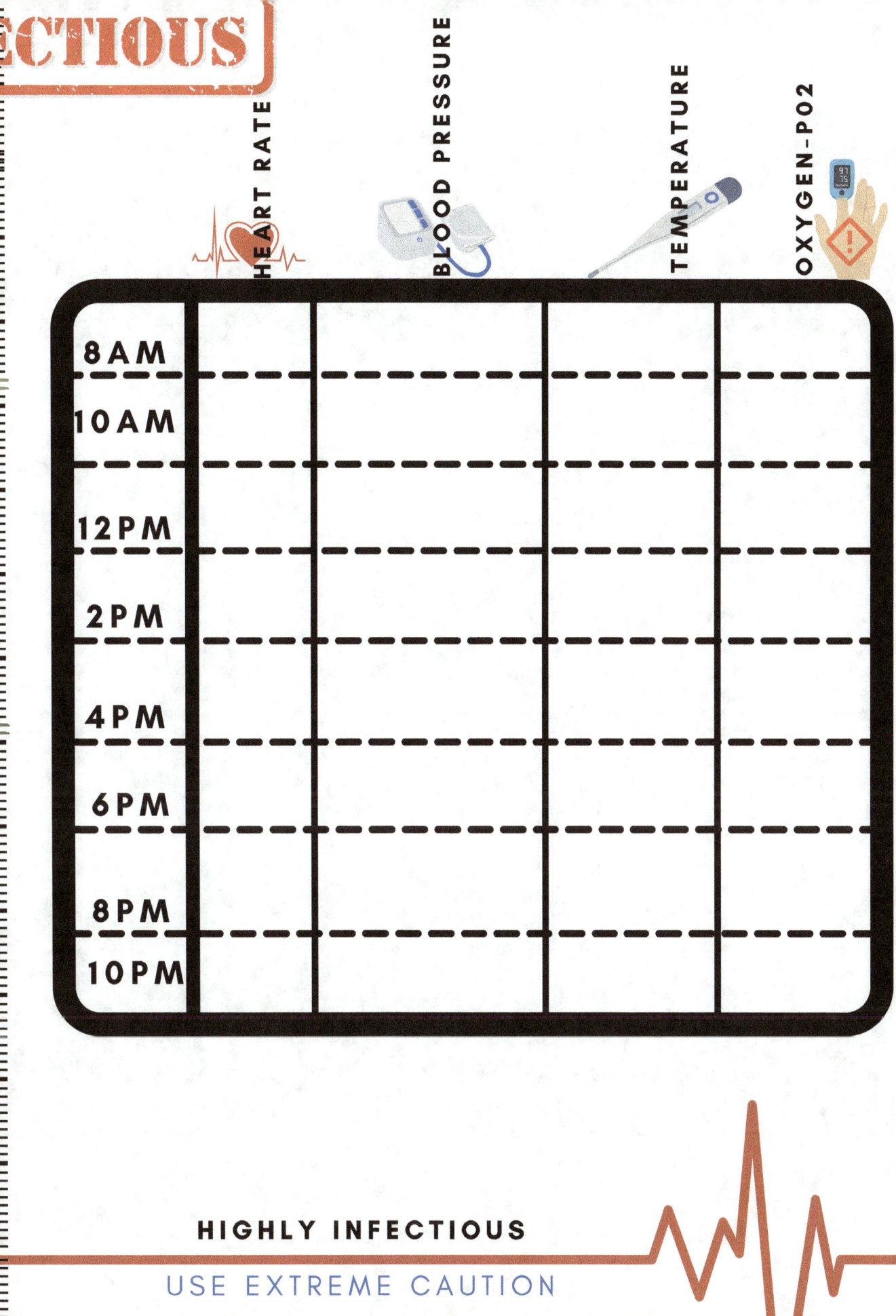

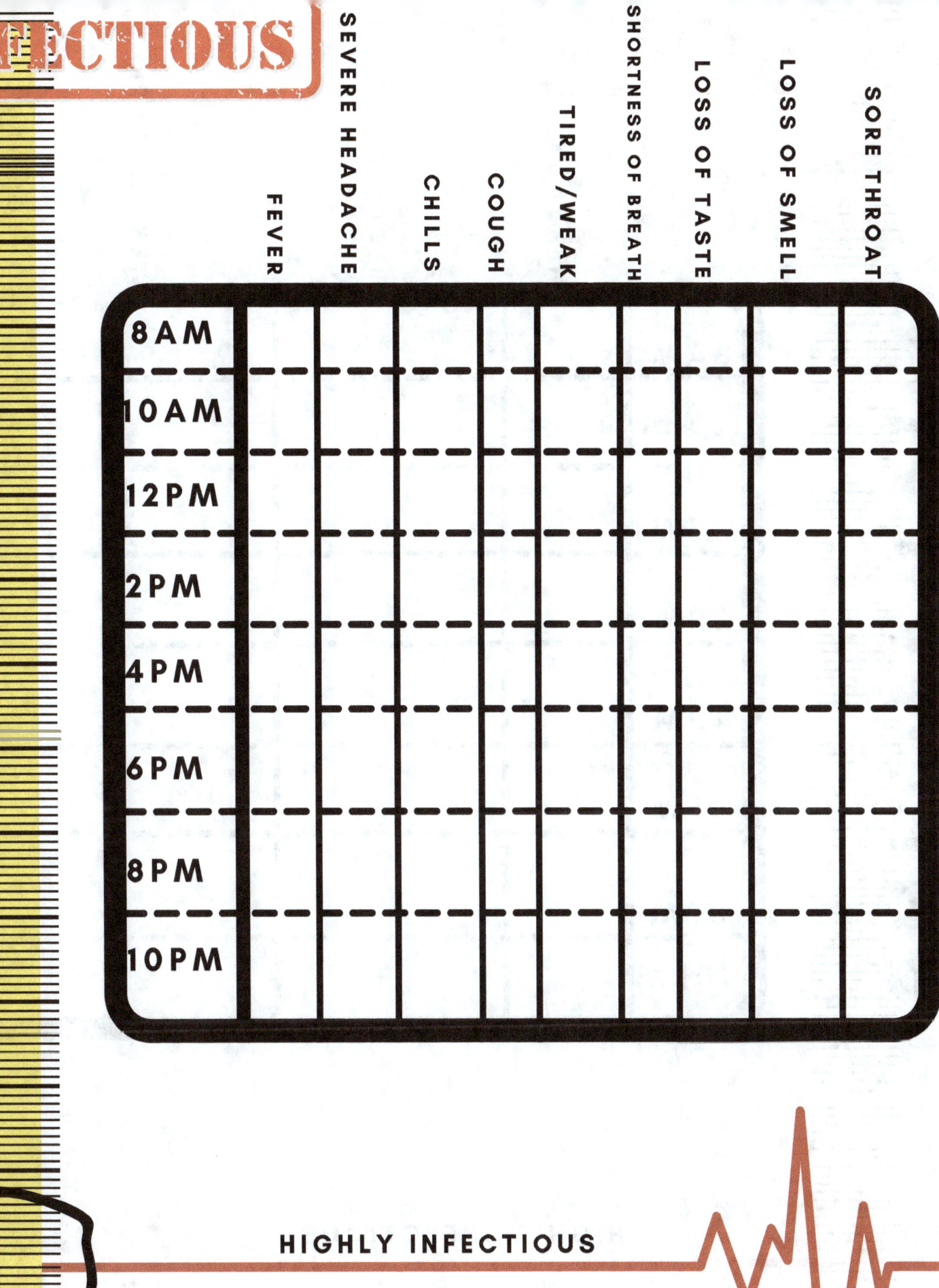

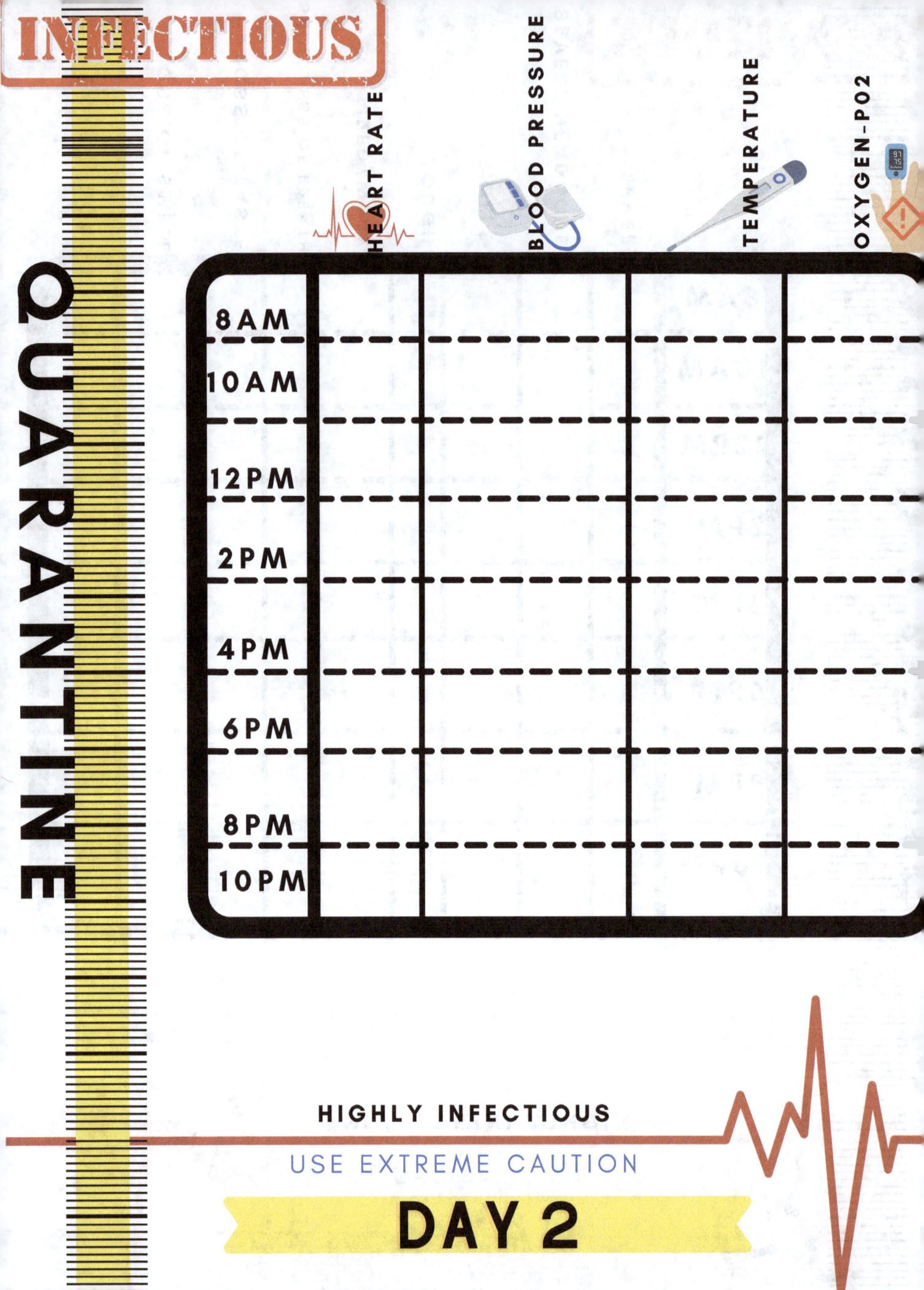

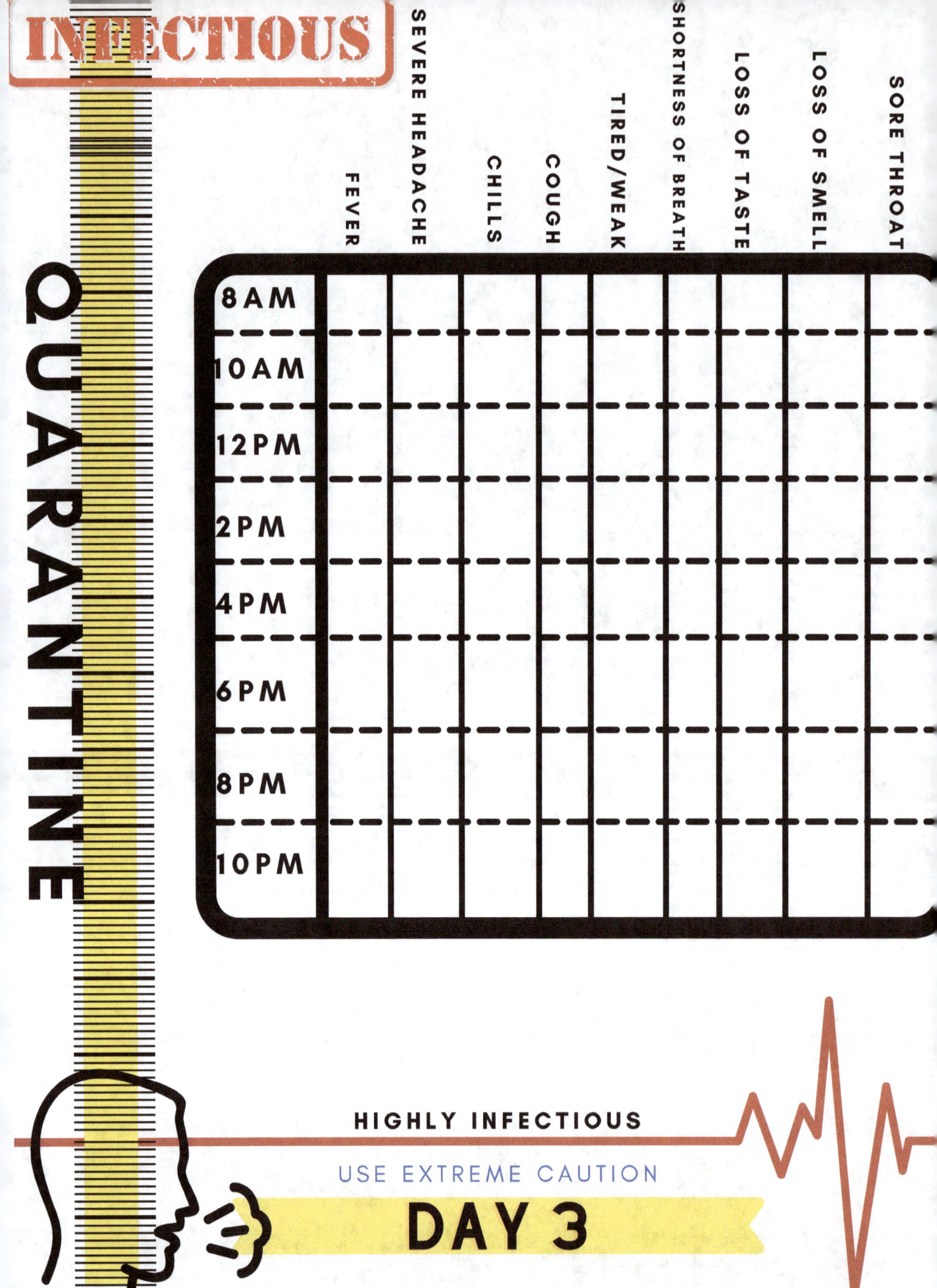

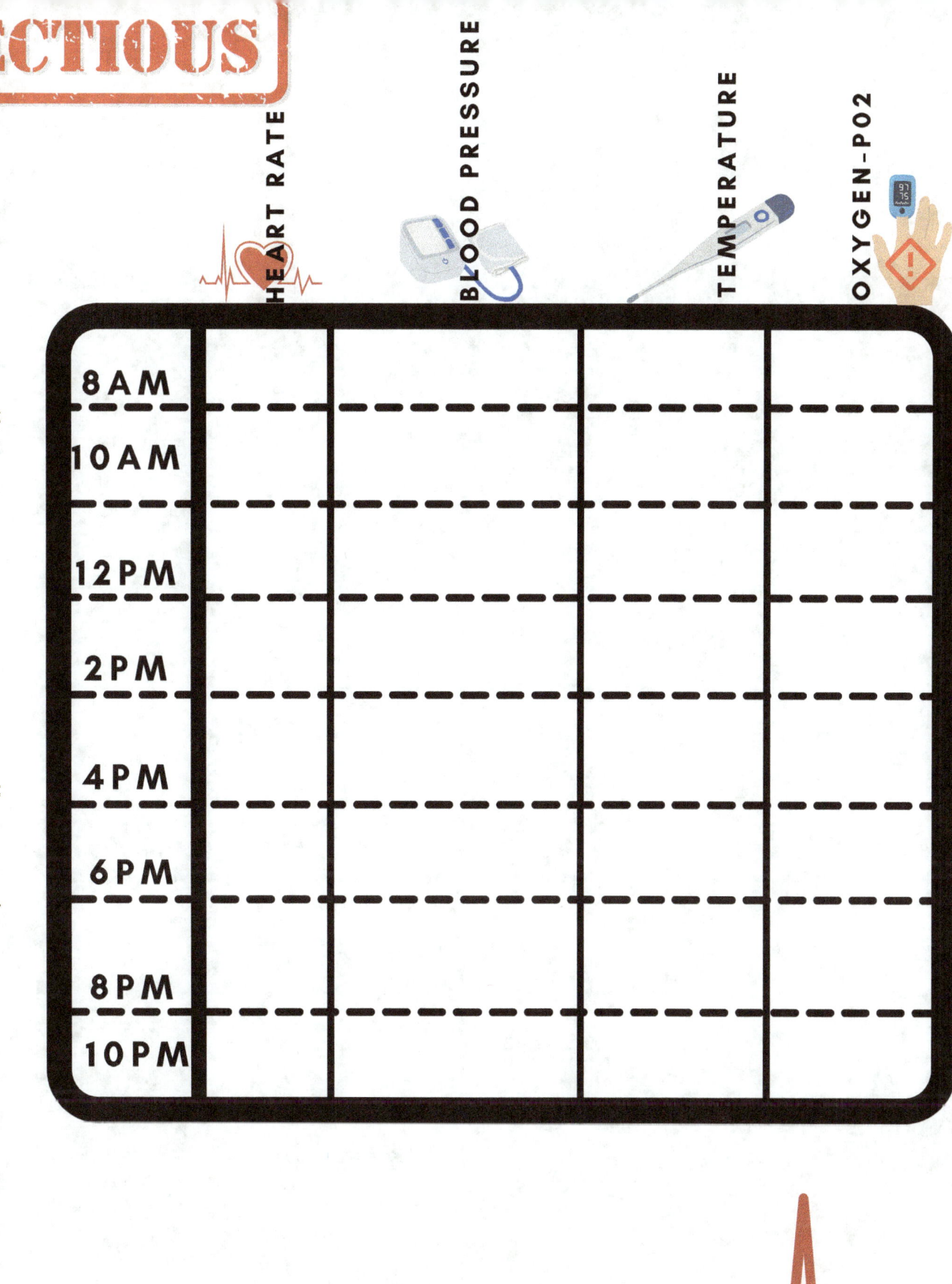

HIGHLY INFECTIOUS

USE EXTREME CAUTION

DAY 3

INFECTIOUS

	FEVER	SEVERE HEADACHE	CHILLS	COUGH	TIRED/WEAK	SHORTNESS OF BREATH	LOSS OF TASTE	LOSS OF SMELL	SORE THROAT
8 AM									
10 AM									
12 PM									
2 PM									
4 PM									
6 PM									
8 PM									
10 PM									

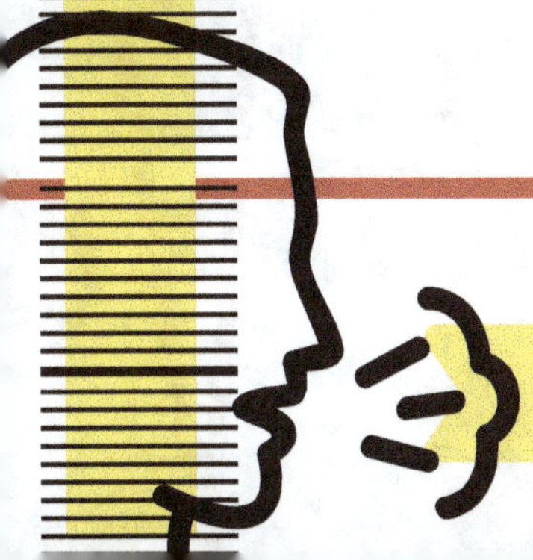

HIGHLY INFECTIOUS

USE EXTREME CAUTION

DAY 4

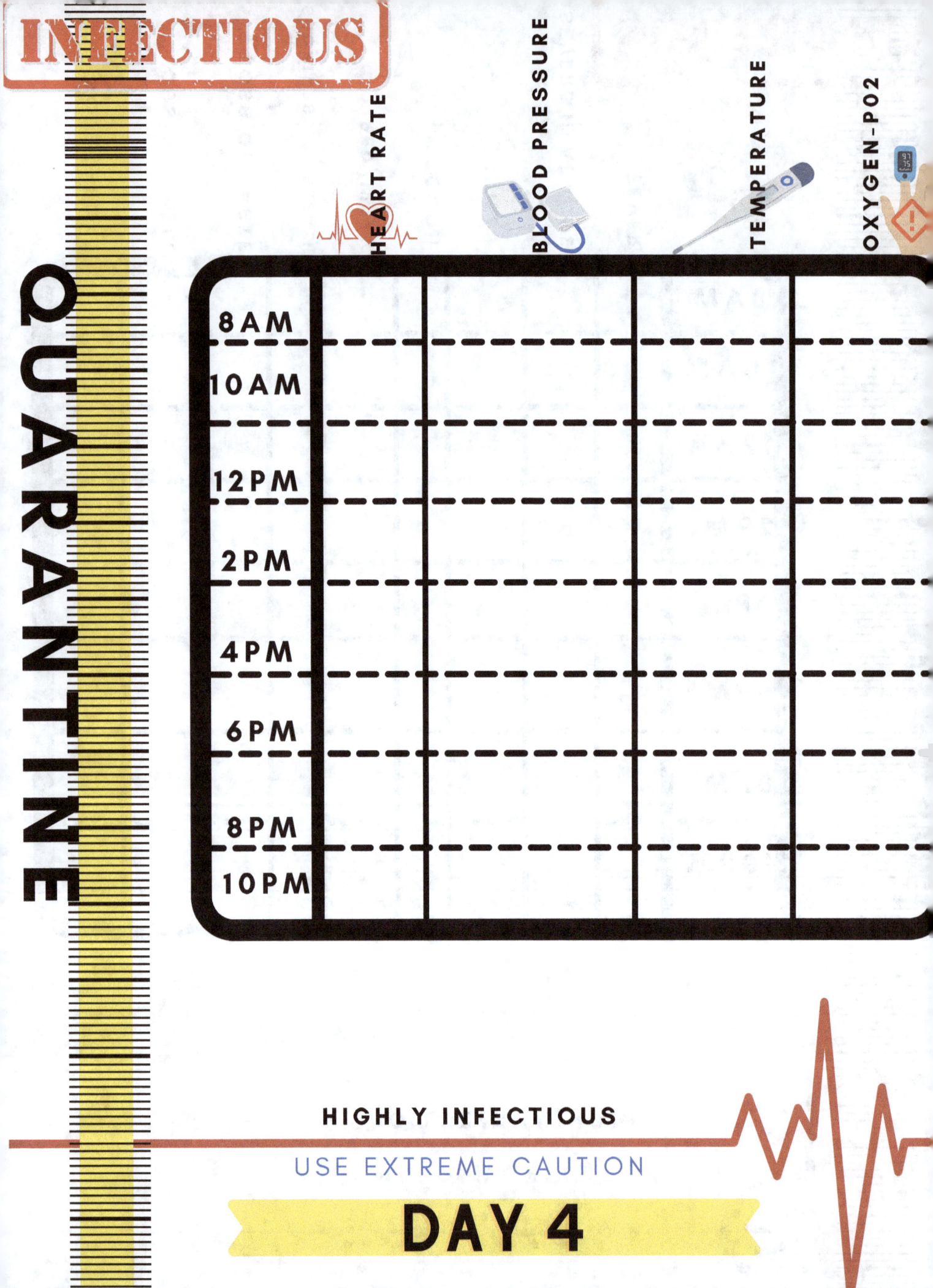

CONTAGIOUS

USE

CAUTION

QUARANTINE

DAYS 5-7

PLACE ON DOOR

QUARANTINE

USE CAUTION

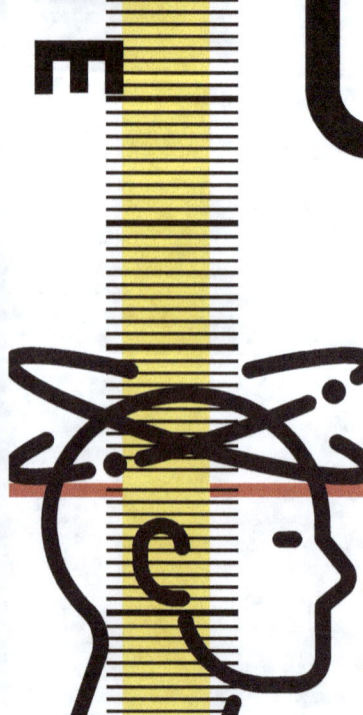

CONTAGIOUS

USE CAUTION

DAYS 5-7

CONTAGIOUS

QUARANTINE

SYMPTOMS & VITAL SIGNS WORKSHEETS

DAYS 5-7

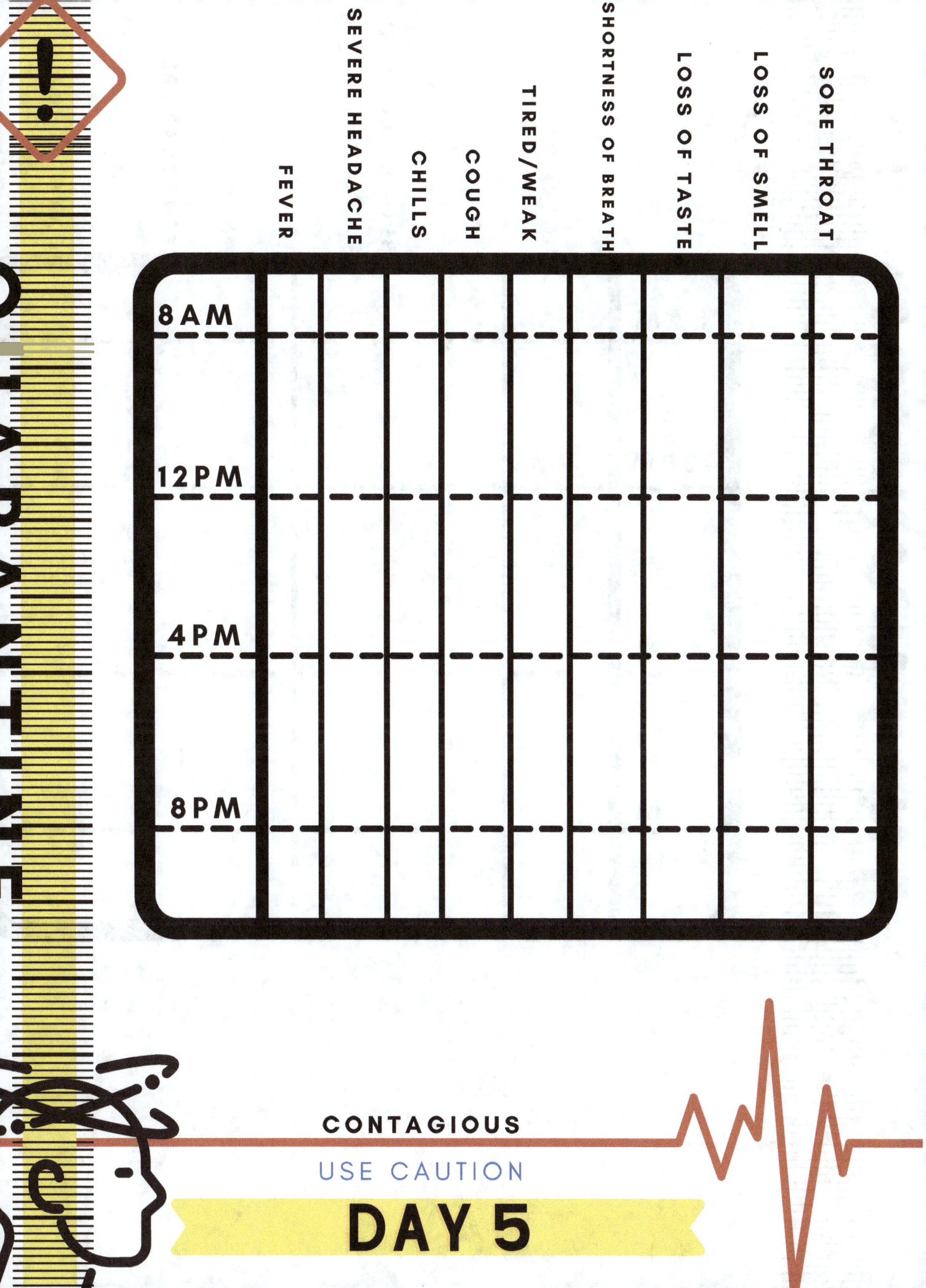

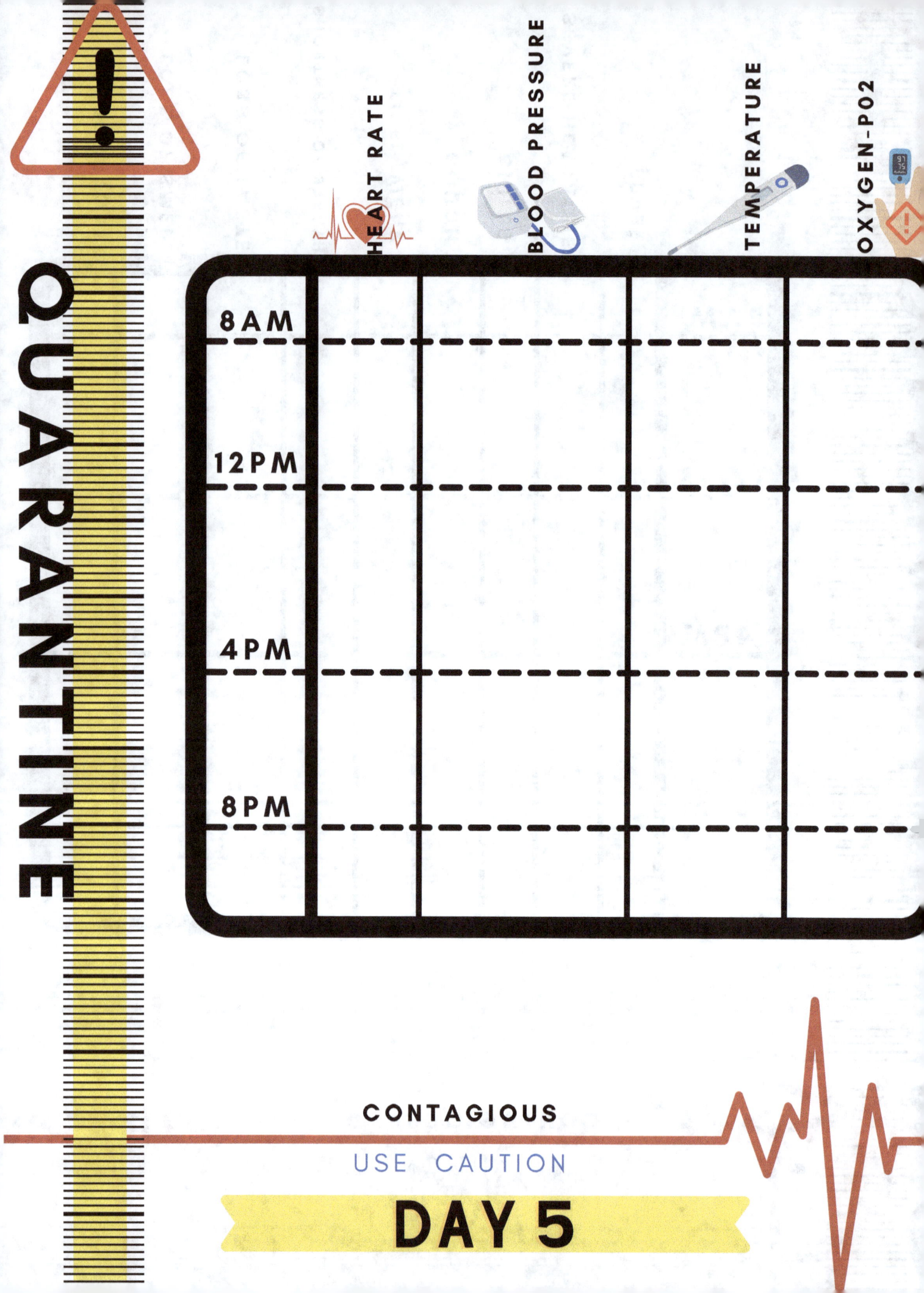

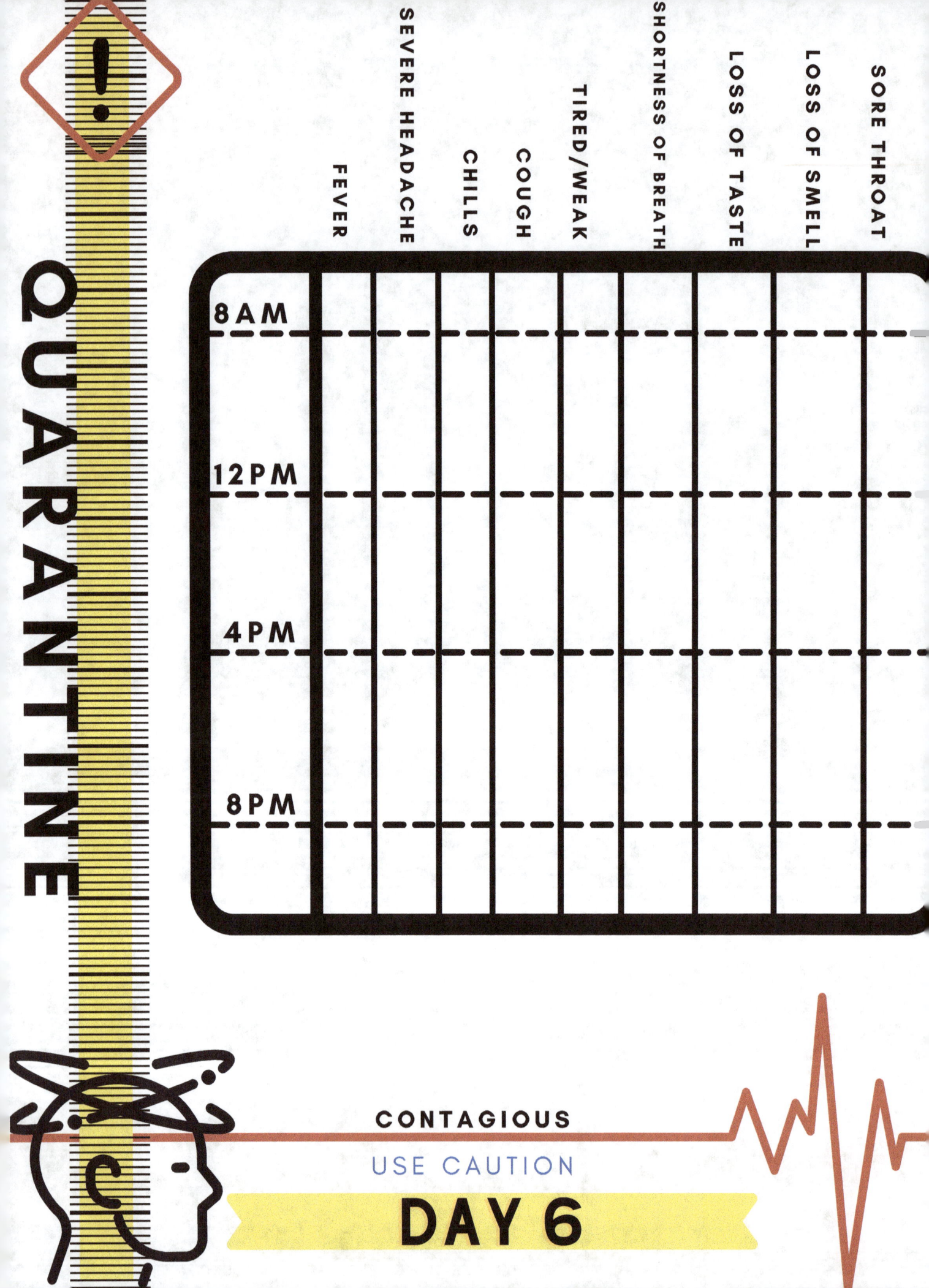

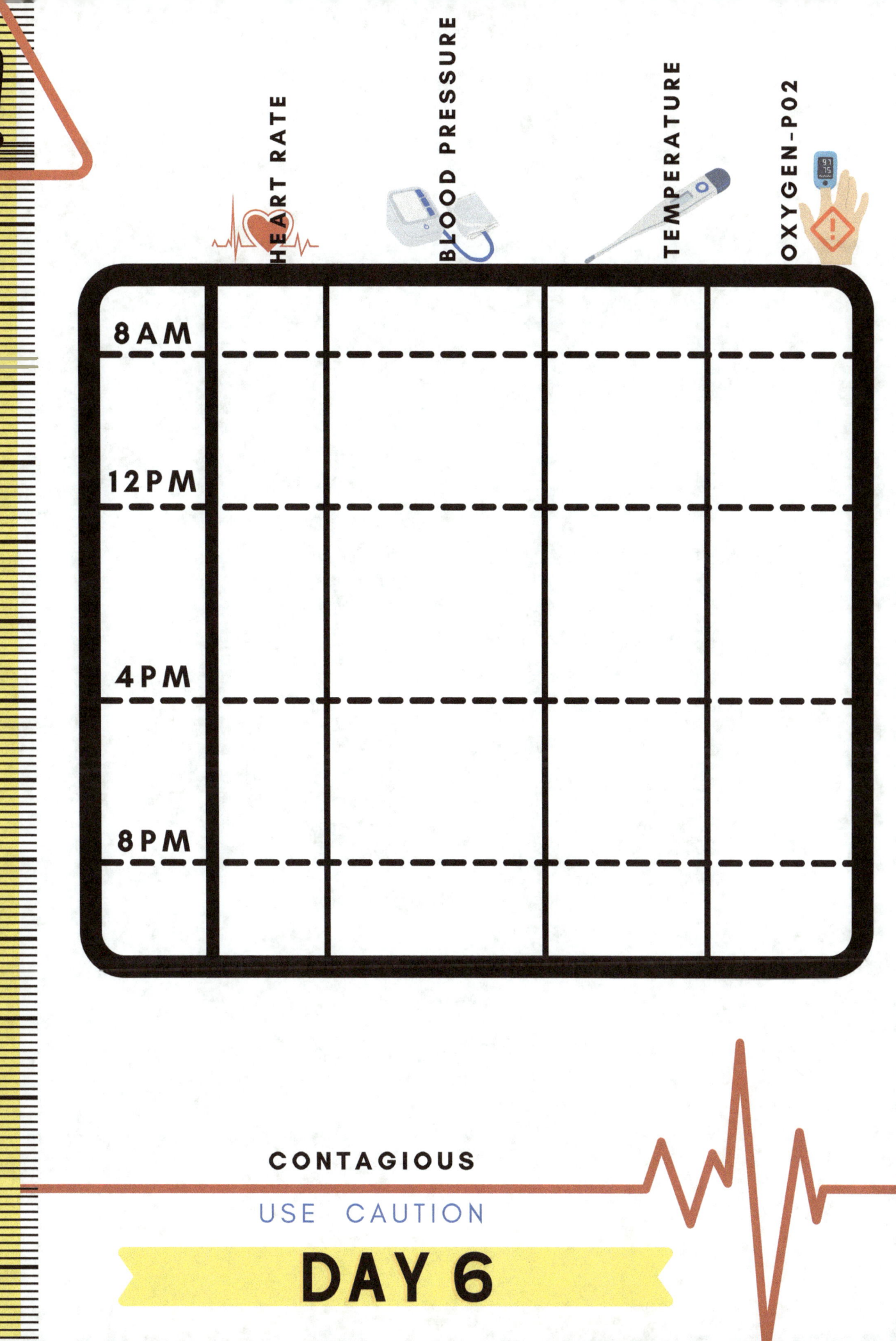

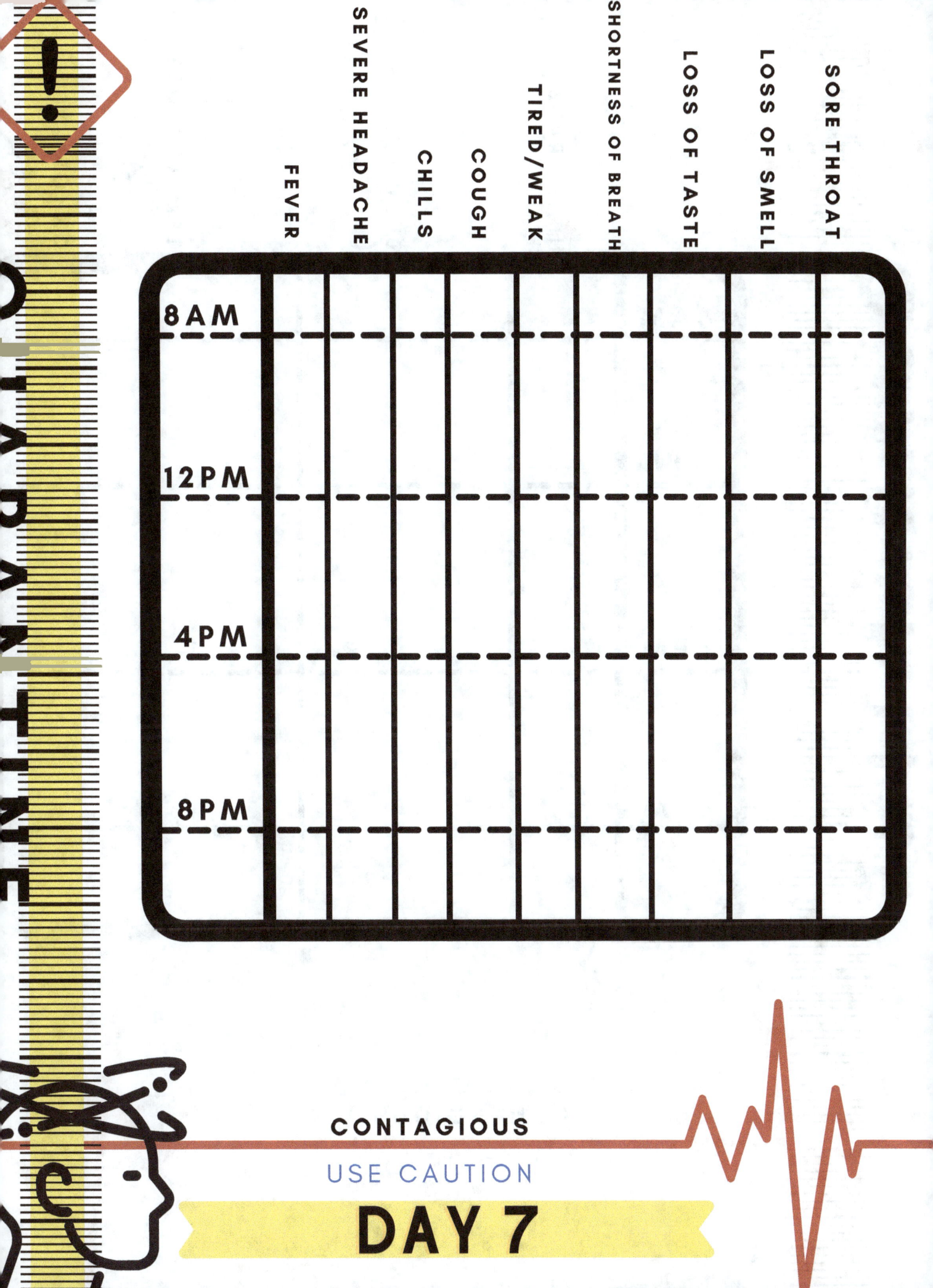

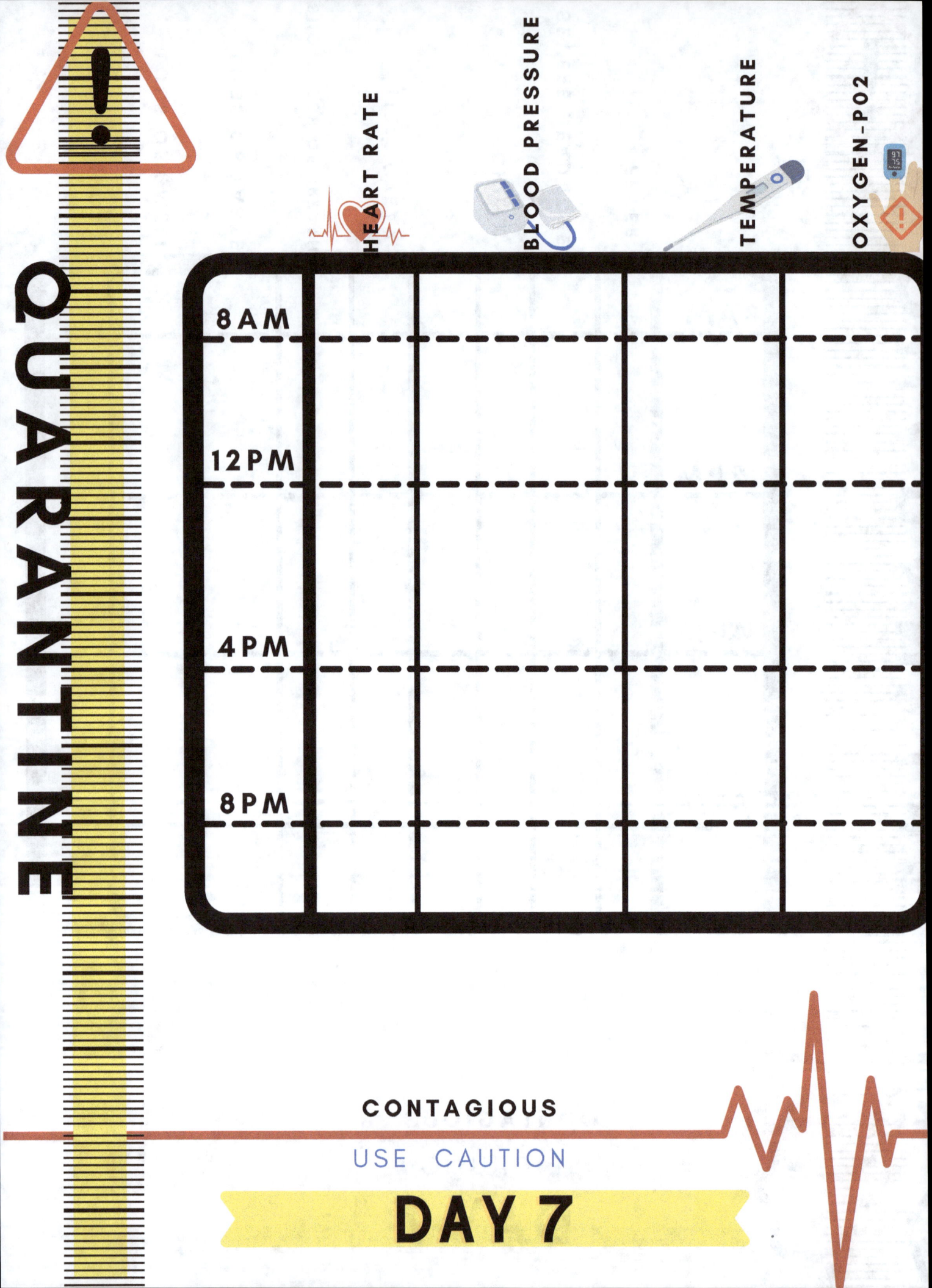

QUARANTINE

AT RISK

MASK UP

DAYS 8-10

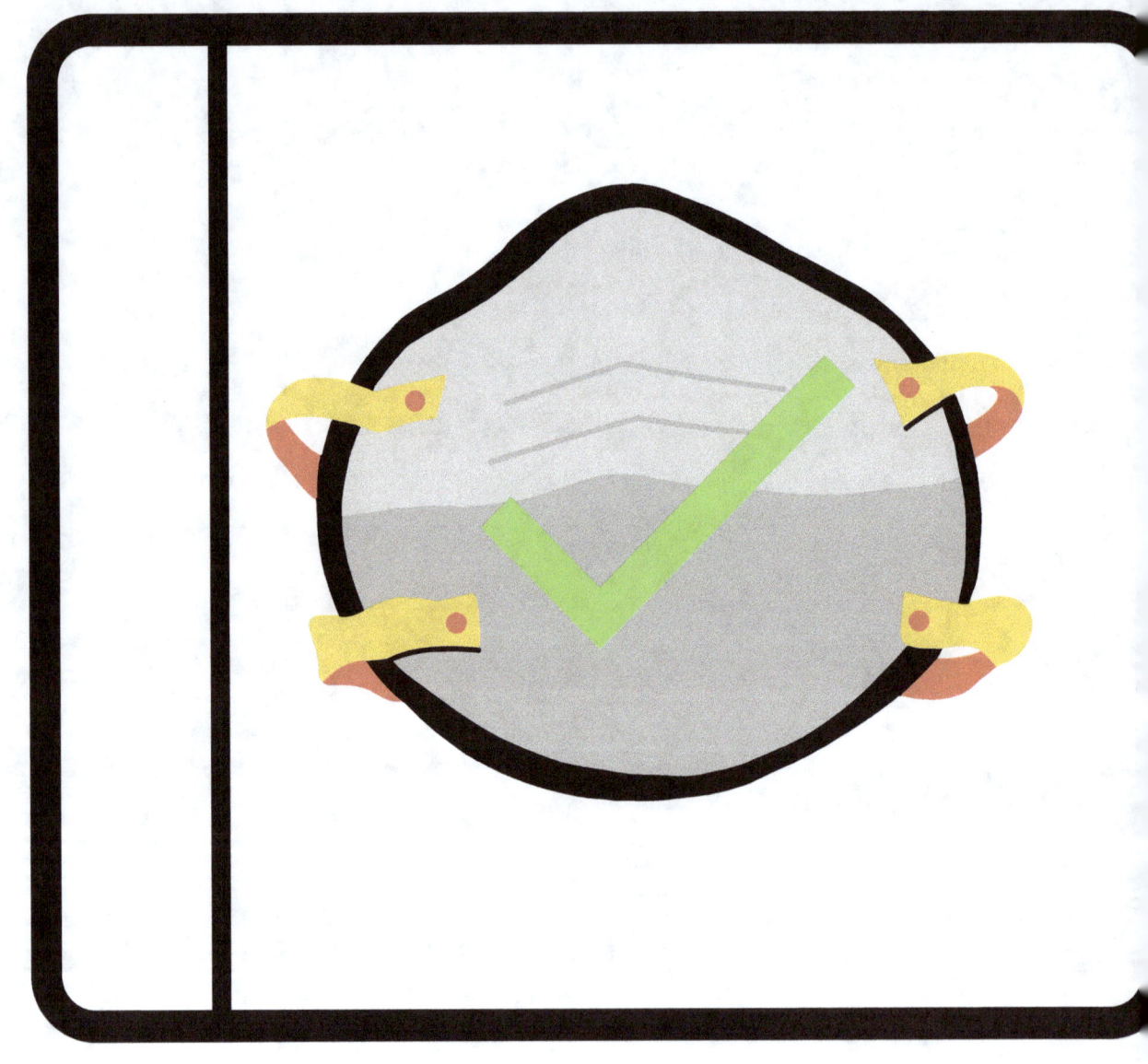

AT RISK

SYMPTOMS & VITAL SIGNS WORKSHEETS

QUARANTINE

DAYS 8-10

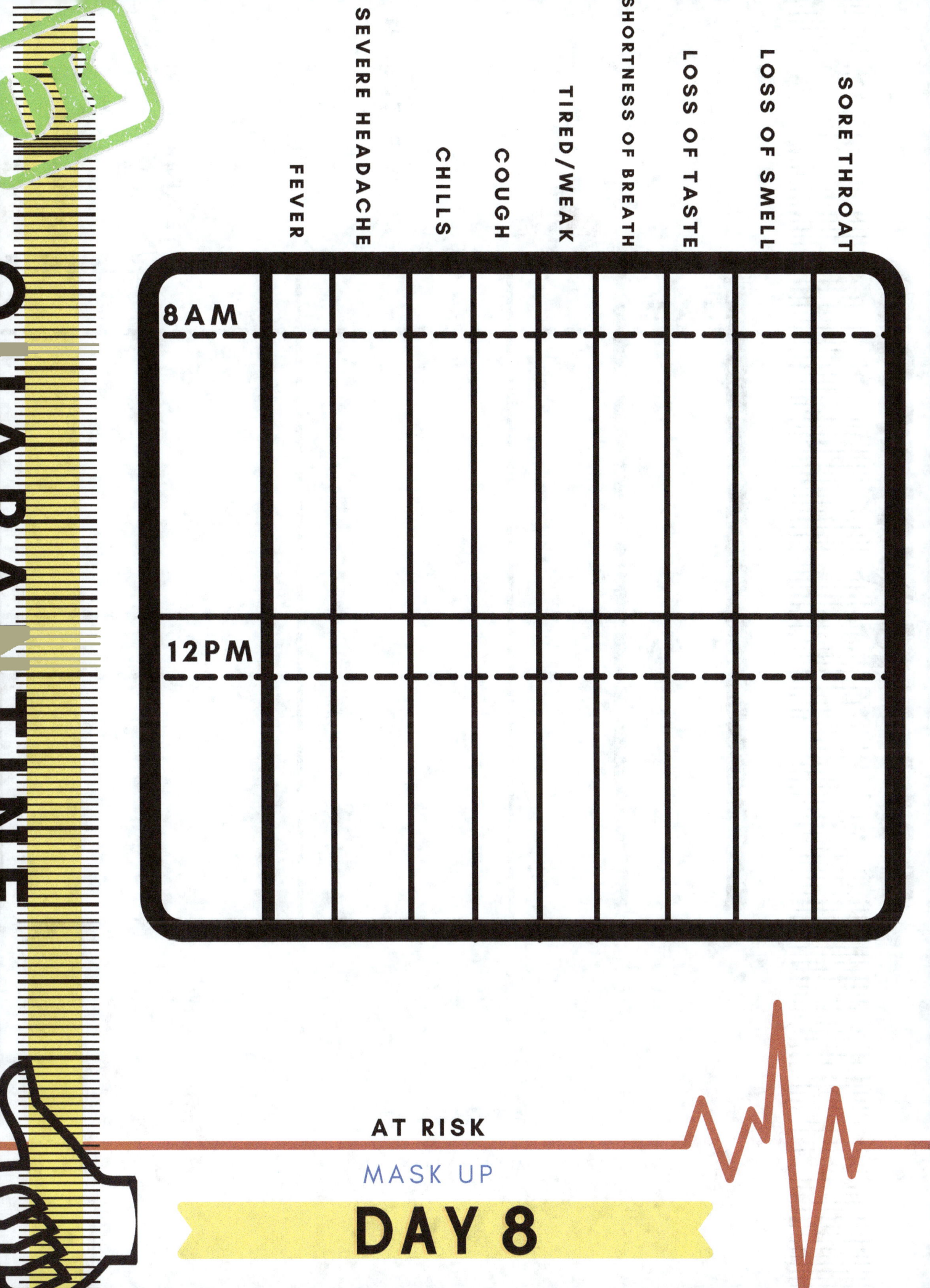

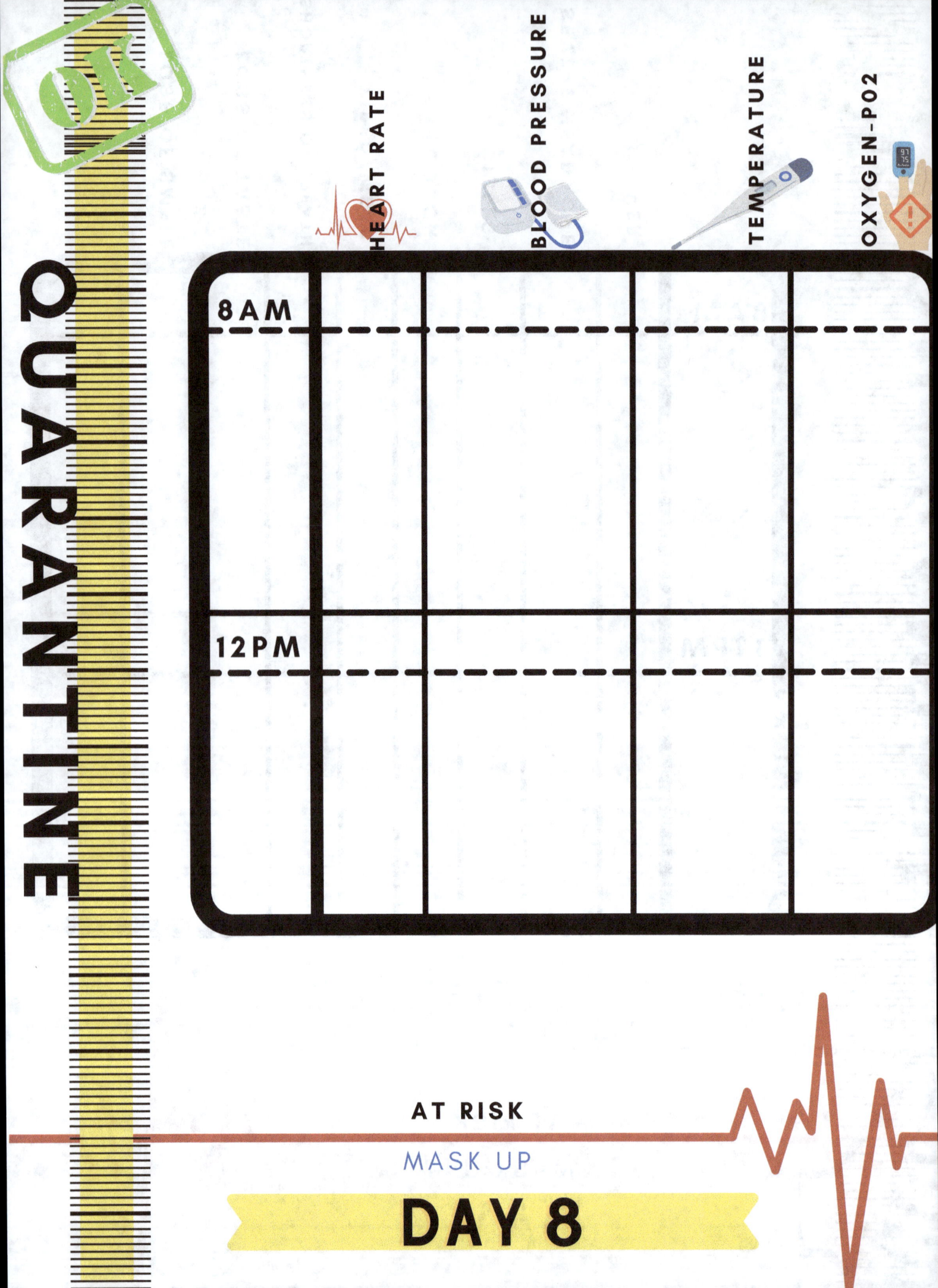

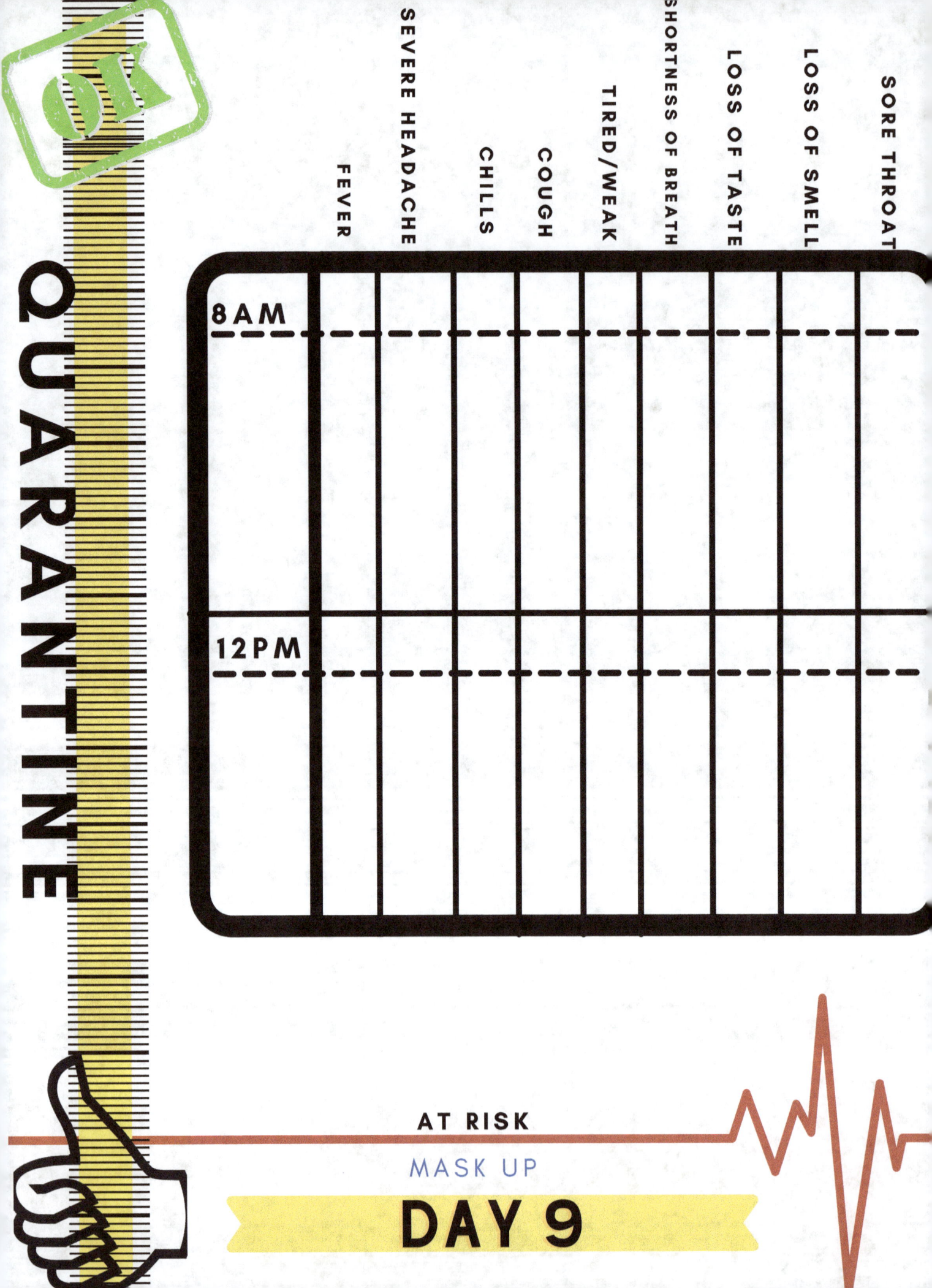

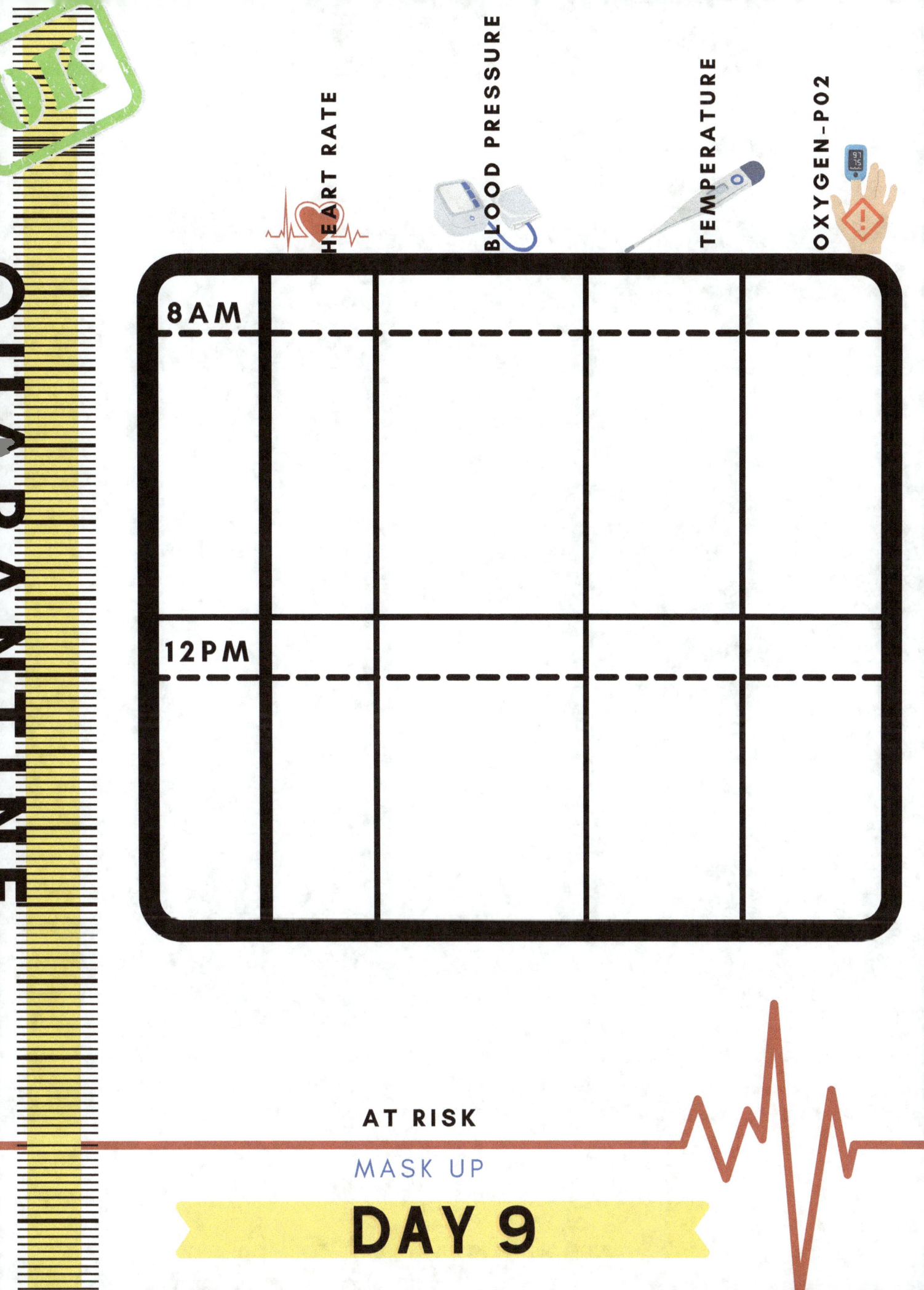

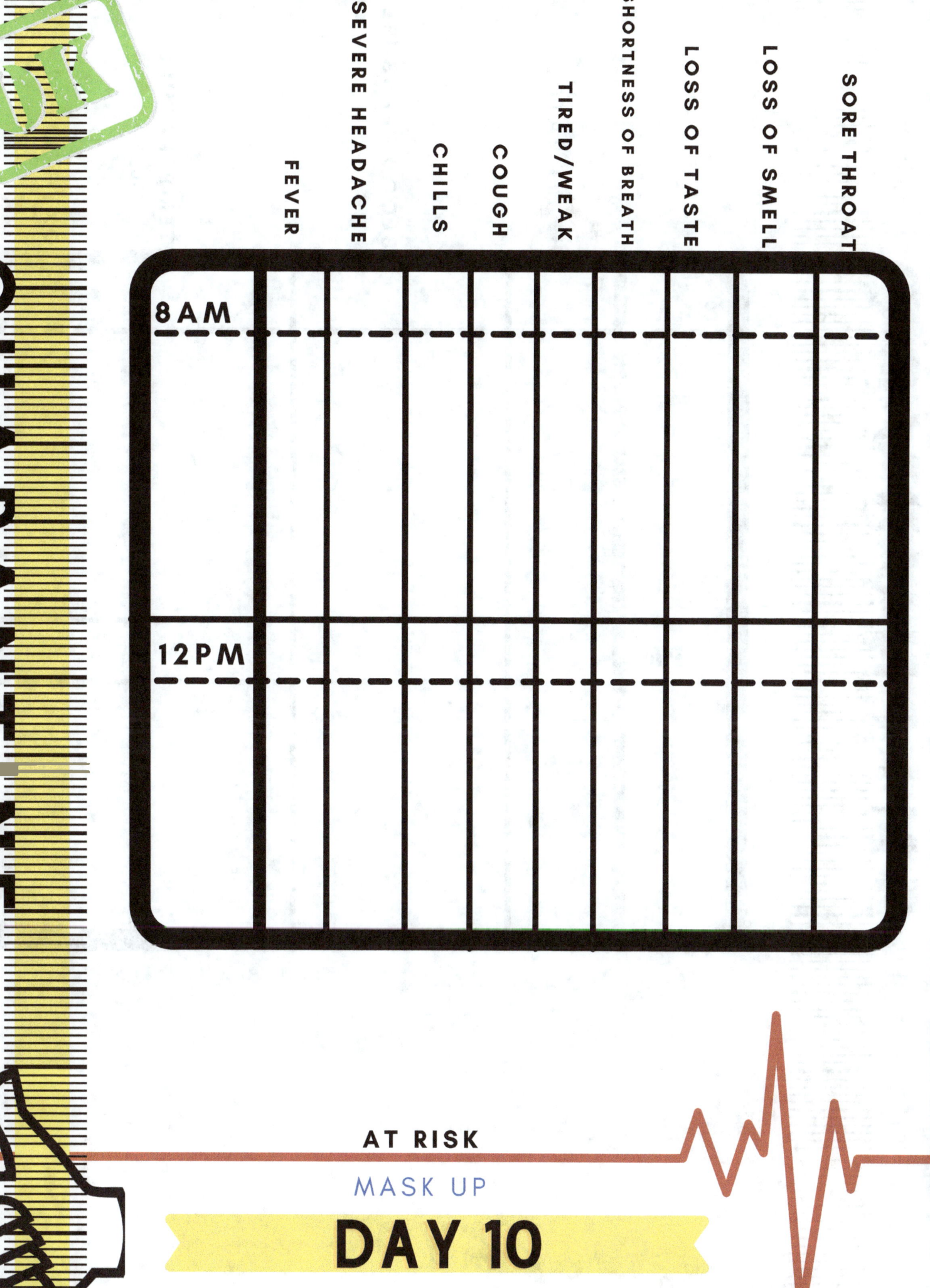

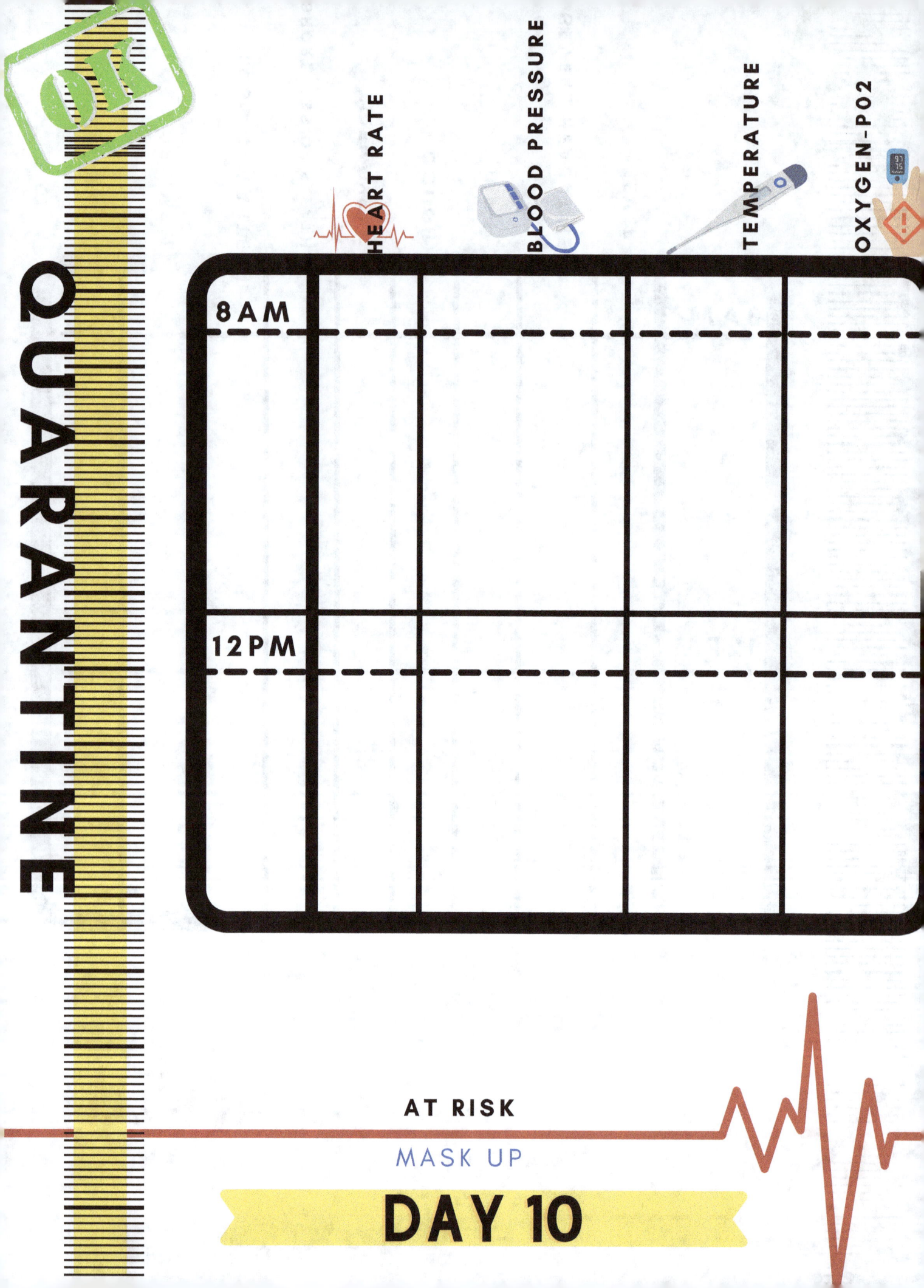

Post Quarantine Mental Recovery

Helping Yourself through Depression

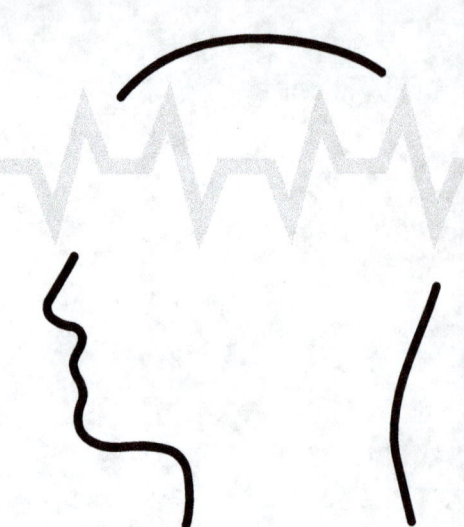

Seek Help From a Trusted Source

Meditate Daily

Read and Speak Positive Affirmations Over Yourself

Express Yourself By Writing Thoughts In A Journal

EXPRESS YOURSELF

EXPRESS YOURSELF

EXPRESS YOURSELF

EXPRESS YOURSELF

EXPRESS YOURSELF

EXPRESS YOURSELF

EXPRESS YOURSELF

EXPRESS YOURSELF

MY THOUGHTS

MY THOUGHTS

MY THOUGHTS

MY THOUGHTS

MY THOUGHTS

MY THOUGHTS

MY THOUGHTS

MY THOUGHTS

MY THOUGHTS

MY THOUGHTS

MY THOUGHTS

MY THOUGHTS

MY THOUGHTS

MY THOUGHTS

www.ingramcontent.com/pod-product-compliance
Lightning Source LLC
Chambersburg PA
CBHW081613220526
45468CB00010B/2853